I0427127

Sirtfood Diet Meal Plan Cookbook

Top Secret Recipes You'll Need for Activate Your Skinny Gene

With Sirtuin Foods.

(The Complete Guide for Beginners)

By: Haley Joseph

Table of Contents

Introduction

It is unfortunate that many people find it easier to complete their tasks for the day than to invest time in cooking healthy meals. This results in a reliance on ready to eat meals or ordering in (mostly junk food.) This may definitely save you time, but you pay a much higher price for this in the long run. Your bad eating habits lead to health complications such as obesity, diabetes, heart diseases, inflammation, and much more.

As per research, over 650 million adults across the world are obese. If you are reading this book, there is a good chance you want to learn to keep your weight under control. The best way to tackle your weight issues is by eating right and having an active lifestyle. Your diet plays a major part in your weight loss journey. To achieve weight loss, you have to focus 80% of your diet and 20% on exercise.

When most people hear the word diet, it usually brings a bad taste in their mouth as they associate diet with eating extremely small portions, drab and tasteless food, and eliminating one food group from their daily food list. All this may not guarantee lasting results, anyway. Well, that's far from the truth. There are many diets out there that allow you to eat a lot of tasty food, not count your calories, and also improve your overall health. One such diet is the sirtfood diet.

If you are struggling to maintain the ideal weight or lose weight, then the sirtfood diet is for you. The Sirtfood diet is an eating protocol that comes in two phases and usually lasts for a month. You will start seeing positive results within the first week of following the diet. Post the four weeks of this diet; you may choose to continue with the cycle for lasting results.

Principles of the Diet

The Sirtfood diet was developed by Glen Matten and Aidan Goggins, famous authors, and nutrition consultants. Their objective was to develop an easy to follow healthy eating pattern that didn't just focus on weight loss alone but also offered overall health benefits. The duo went on the sirtfood diet by eating sirtuin rich foods in their everyday meals and discovered the secret and healing powers of the sirtfood diet.

The sirtfood diet relies on a simple theory of consuming sirtuin rich foods. Sirtuins are a protein compound that regulates various body functions such as metabolism, inflammation, and cell building. A few plant compounds are rich in these sirtuin protein compounds, and they are called sirtfoods.

The Sirtfood diet enables you to eat things such as dark chocolate, red wine, cruciferous vegetables, walnuts, matcha green tea, etc. These are not just desirable, but also help activate the skinny gene pathways in your body. These skinny genes mimic the effects of fasting and exercise, so you can eat a full meal and not have to train or exercise intensively to reap the weight loss benefits.

There is much to be learned about the sirtfood diet, and this book has all the information you need to know. You will learn about the benefits of the diet and how it uses the skinny gene to help you lose weight. You will also learn about the two phases of the diet and the sirtfoods that you will need to include in your diet. This book also comes with numerous sirtfood recipes, which are easy to make. These recipes are extremely nutritious and tasty and rich in sirtfood certified ingredients that will help you lose weight while eating.

Before you plan to make the switch, remember that it is not easy to switch to any diet overnight, so give yourself some time. Learn to be kind to yourself, especially as your body adapts to the changes in your diet. Notice the signs your body gives you and see how far you can push yourself. If you take it slow, before you know it, you will easily transition to the sirtfood diet and reap the many benefits it offers.

If you are keen to learn more about this diet, let's start without further delay.

Chapter 1:
What is the Sirtfood Diet?

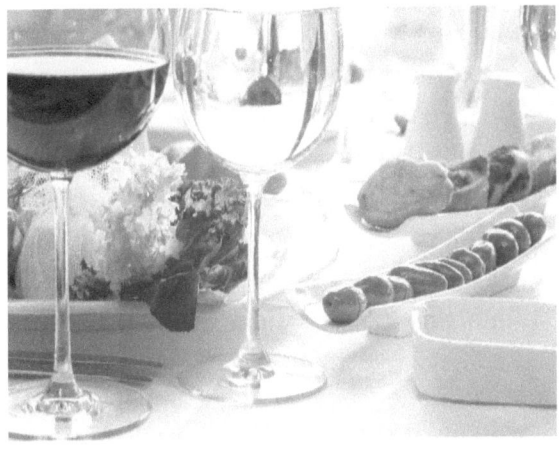

Fasting has proven to be beneficial for weight loss. The creators of the diet, Glen Matten and Aidan Goggins, were inspired by the idea of fasting when they developed the sirtfood diet. The sirtfood diet benefits your body in the same way fasting does, but it does not require you to fast. Yes, you heard that right. You can reap the benefits of fasting without actively fasting.

Before we understand how that works, let us look at the theory this diet is based on.

Sirtfood Diet Theory

The sirtfood diet is not exactly a diet, but an eating pattern to help you lead a healthier life. You can enjoy the benefits of fasting without depriving your body of the food and nutrition it needs. Fasting as a concept has existed since the beginning of civilization, but it is not an easy practice to follow. It is unfortunate that many people punish their bodies by following arduous fasting diets and eating patterns just to lose weight as fast as possible. If followed holistically, it can benefit the body, but most people take extreme measures for fast results, which can lead to issues such as inadequate nutrition, imbalance in blood sugar, anemia, fatigue, and a weakened immune system.

Most people do not understand that fasting diets work well because they activate the skinny gene in your body. When this gene is triggered, it does not allow your body to store fat. Your body automatically shifts into survival mode when you do not consume enough food to provide it with energy. When you reduce your caloric intake, your body targets the fat reserves to provide the cells and organs with energy. What the Sirtfood diet does is it essentially provides the benefits of fasting and activates your skinny gene without having to punish your body through the arduous fasting.

Understanding the Sirtfood Diet

Matten and Goggins developed this diet while they worked at a private gym. They are well-known nutritionists and health consultants who have been in the industry for a long. According to them, the skinny gene in your body can help you lose weight if you eat the right foods to trigger it. The sirtfood diet only includes foods that are rich in a compound called sirtuins. Sirtuins are protein compounds that benefit the body in numerous ways. The benefits of sirtuins are:

- Regulate different functions in the body

- Reduce inflammation

- Increase lifespan

- Improve metabolism

The duo believed different plant compounds could help increase the sirtuins in your body. These sirtuin rich foods are called sirtfoods, and we will look at some of these foods in detail in the third chapter. Unlike fasting, the sirtfood diet requires you to eat healthy and wholesome meals made with sirtfood rich ingredients, which release the protein compound in your body. This ensures you provide your body with the required nutrition. Also, you have to restrict your caloric intake for the first week in order to activate your skinny gene, which also helps to reduce weight in a healthy manner.

According to the author duo who designed this diet, the sirtfood diet reduces the risk of various diseases and also activates the skinny gene. Since the diet is still relatively new, there is limited research available to back this statement, although a host of celebrities such as Adele, David Haye, and Jodie Kidd who followed this diet showed tremendous results.

The foods that increase your sirtuin compounds have many healthy properties and come with a host of benefits. A lot of the foods on the list are also considered to be superfoods. Both Matten and

Goggins performed intensive tests to understand how the diet affects people. They conducted these trials and tests at their fitness center on 39 subjects and published their study's details and findings in a book they co-authored. The study's objective was to consume only sirtfoods and determine how a person's body changes due to these ingredients.

The subjects were required to perform little exercise every day to aid weight loss and muscle growth. Their weight was monitored regularly; Matten and Goggins noted that some people also developed muscle mass. The duo continued to monitor their subjects' weight even after they went back to their earlier lifestyle. They noted most people were able to maintain their weight as long as they managed their caloric intake.

It is important to note that when you deprive your body of calories, your body attacks stored glycogen to produce energy before it attacks the fat stores. Therefore, when you are on any diet, the weight you lose during the first few weeks is mostly water and glycogen. Your body needs four molecules of water to store one molecule of glucose, and these molecules are the first to be attacked when there is a calorie deficit.

Matten and Goggins noted that subjects who went back to their old eating patterns gained the weight they lost and more in a span of a week. Only those who continued to follow the principles of the diet and consumed sirtuin-rich foods continued to lose weight. The sirtfood diet will help you lose weight in the first few weeks as you change your entire eating pattern and consume more sirtuin rich foods. If you choose to go back to your old eating patterns, the weight will come back. You can only maintain your weight if you continue to follow this eating pattern.

As mentioned earlier, the sirtfood diet increases your intake of foods rich in sirtuins. This, coupled with the calorie restriction prescribed by the diet, offers its weight loss benefits. Sirtuins stimulate the production of a specific protein known as Anaplastic Lymphoma Kinase (ALK). This is believed to be responsible for the weight loss associated with this diet. The skinny gene is responsible for regulating the production of ALK. The primary difference in our metabolism is responsible for one's ability to lose or gain weight. For instance, some struggle to lose weight while others face difficulty-gaining weight. A group of scientists set out to determine the primary reason for this difference. During their research, they stumbled upon what they call the skinny gene.

The presence of a variant of the ALK gene regulates an individual's ability to gain weight regardless of their diet. The researchers established the same. This gene is present in a part of the brain responsible for regulating appetite, known as the hypothalamus. The skinny gene also regulates the fat stored within the body and the intake of fats. Scientists observed the DNA of more than 45,000 individuals. They also used data from the Estonia biobank, a massive biological database. During their research, the scientist discovered individuals with any variant of this specific gene had a tough time gaining weight. If weight loss is your priority, activating this gene is a good idea. The simplest way to do this is by following the sirtfood diet.

Benefits of the Sirtfood Diet

The diet's creators conducted several trials and studies to determine the effect of sirtfoods on their subjects. They noted every participant lost at least seven pounds at the end of the first week. The participants also claimed they slept better, were more alert, and had clear skin after they began the diet. They also claimed that the various sirtfoods included in this diet satiated their appetite and curbed their hunger. These foods had the nutrients needed to improve your body's metabolism, which helped with weight loss.

The duo also believed that sirtfoods had a better chance of reducing cardiovascular and other chronic illnesses and diseases since they improved the functioning of the immune system. Some participants in the study had heart diseases, diabetes, and Alzheimer's. They noted these participants showed reduced symptoms of these diseases when they switched to the sirtfood diet.

Matten and Goggins also mentioned the diet could improve your body's metabolism by reversing any persisting issues. This can only happen if you follow the diet in the long term. They also believed this diet is an eating pattern and a way of life since it helps people stay healthy and fit. The creators noted from their studies that most participants did not lose muscle, although they lost weight.

Chapter 2:
Phases of the Diet

You now know what the Sirtfood diet is and the benefits it offers. There is a lot of research being conducted to learn more about what the diet can do for you. It is important to learn more about the process of this diet before you begin. This chapter sheds some light on the phases of the diet.

The diet is broken down into two phases, and each phase has a set of instructions you need to follow if you want to change the way your body reacts to these foods. If you want the sirtuins to work for you, make sure you stick to the diet's patterns. Stick to the principles of the diet if you want your metabolism to change. The two phases of this diet last between one and three weeks. You can continue to repeat the phases of this diet until you meet your fitness and weight-loss objectives.

You need to prepare yourself before you begin the Sirtfood diet. The diet is not restrictive, but there are some foods you need to include in your diet. For example, you need to drink green juices regularly when you switch to this diet. Let us first look at the phases of the diet before we look at the sirtfood compliant food list.

Hyper Success Stage

The first phase, also known as the hyper success stage, requires you to reduce your caloric intake from the usual to 800 – 1000 calories per day. This stage of the diet lasts for seven days, and it is divided into two parts. The first part of this phase lasts for three days. During these three days, you need to stick to the following objectives:

- Drink green juices thrice a day

- Eat one meal rich in sirtfoods

This does not mean you can eat anything you please in your other meals. The first three days of the diet may seem restrictive, but look at the bigger picture. Focus on the benefits of the diet and remember the first part of the phase lasts only three days, which is a very small price to pay.

When the three days are done, you move onto the next part of the phase. In these four days, you can increase your caloric intake to 1000 – 1300 calories. You need to drink green juice twice a day and eat two Sirtfoods rich meals during this part. When you finish this stage, you have to move onto the next phase. Experts state you should continue this phase for at least three weeks to ensure your body adapts to the change in your eating patterns.

However, you can choose to continue phase one for three weeks or move on to the next phase after the seventh day. You will soon notice that you are losing weight because of the caloric restriction. This phase also helps you detoxify. You no longer consume unhealthy foods or pile on excess calories since your meals are filled with healthy sirtfoods. When you succeed with the first phase, you can move onto the second phase of this diet.

Maintenance Phase

The second phase, also known as the maintenance phase, is when you work on your eating pattern and lifestyle to ensure you maintain the benefits you reaped in the previous stage. Unlike the first phase of this diet, which is restrictive, you can eat proper sirtfood rich meals since you no longer have to replace your meals with green juice. In this phase, you need to drink only one glass of green juice. All your other meals have to be Sirtfood rich meals (you can choose the recipes shared in this book for these meals.) This phase lasts for two weeks, but you can extend the phase for longer if you want to. As the name suggests, it is the maintenance stage, and if you continue eating Sirtfood rich meals, you will continue to lose weight or at worse maintain your weight loss.

At this point in the diet, you no longer have to worry about your caloric intake and are allowed to eat wholesome meals. Having said that, you cannot consume too many calories. When you maintain a caloric deficit, your body begins to use the fat stores to produce energy. If you want to reap the benefits of the diet while you maintain your caloric intake, you need to be mindful of the food you eat.

The Sirtfood diet makes you conscious about the foods you consume. You need to stop relying on unhealthy food and replace them with healthier sirtfoods listed in the following chapter. When you change your eating habits, you learn to regulate your intake. Your body also changes how it processes food. If you feel your body needs a boost, restart the phases of the diet. If you want to maintain the benefits of this diet, you need to increase the intake of the foods listed in the chapter below.

Chapter 3:
The Best Sirtfoods

Before we look at the different recipes in the book, you need to understand the different reasons why some foods are included in the Sirtfood diet. This chapter lists some Sirtfood diets and their benefits.

Kale

Most diets include kale since it is considered a superfood. This vegetable is a part of the cabbage family and is low in calories. One cup of kale contains 33 calories, 3 grams of protein, 2 grams of carbs, and 2 grams of fiber. This vegetable is also rich in antioxidants, which reduce any damage caused to the cells due to oxidative stress. Oxidative stress is one of the main reasons for the development of chronic illnesses. The polyphenols and flavonoids are the primary antioxidants in kale.

Capers

Capers, or caper berries, are native to the Mediterranean. Most Mediterranean foods have pickled capers, and this food has fewer calories when compared to most vegetables and fruit. One ounce of capers contains only 6.5 calories and 1 gram of fiber. You can increase your intake of capers without any worry, especially if you want to increase your fiber intake. Dietary fiber helps to stabilize and maintain your blood sugar levels since it controls your body's need to absorb sugar.

Red Wine

As per research by Singh K et al. (2018), resveratrol, an antioxidant, activates sirtuins. The skin of grapes that are used to make wine is high in resveratrol. This compound is also known to aid in weight loss. Resveratrol reduces the risk of heart diseases, diabetes, and aids in weight loss. Therefore, it is not a bad thing to drink a glass of wine with your meals. Having said that, you should drink it in moderation since it can throw your blood sugar off balance.

Dark Chocolate

As per a study conducted by Bohannon J et al. (2015), chocolate can help in weight loss. However, it is best to eat cocoa nibs or dark chocolate since these do not contain milk solids and added sugars. Research also shows that dark chocolate contains antioxidants and other compounds that reduce the risk of cardiovascular diseases. These compounds also improve your mood and mental abilities. If you cannot control your chocolate intake, you do not have to worry because the Sirtfood diet does not restrict your intake of dark chocolate. Another study conducted by Duarte D et al. (2015) suggests that cocoa and dark chocolate are associated with improving the body's ability to activate the sirtuin pathway.

Red Onion

Red onions are used in different cuisines, and it is a versatile ingredient. It is low in calories and can be added to most dishes without any worry. Slavin J et al. (2007) conducted a study that showed that red onions contain enough fiber to help people maintain their weight. Quercetin, a flavonoid found in red onion, aids in weight loss. This flavonoid also improves the functioning of the skinny gene in your body by activating the sirtuins, which helps you lose weight easily.

Strawberries

If you love strawberries, then this diet is perfect for you. This berry is not only delicious but also is rich in nutrients. One cup of strawberries has fewer calories than most berries. It only contains 50 calories and 3 grams of dietary fiber. This berry also helps you meet at least 30% and 45% of your required intake of manganese and Vitamin C. You can easily eat a bowl of strawberries as a snack, but most people use this fruit when they make desserts, with added sugar, processed flour, and dairy produce, which doesn't offer any benefits to your body. Some other vitamins and minerals present in strawberries are potassium, ellagitannins, pelargonidin, folate, ellagic acid, and procyanidins. Strawberries, like grapes, are rich in resveratrol, which is an anti-inflammatory ingredient.

Extra Virgin Olive Oil

Extra virgin olive oil is used in most Mediterranean and Italian dishes. This oil is known for its benefits and is extracted from one of the oldest known trees cultivated in the world. People have used olive oil for over 9000 years, and it was used as a key ingredient in most traditional medicines and medicinal pastes. Hippocrates, the Father of medicine, also suggested that this oil could cure almost any disease. This oil is extracted from the olive fruit and is the purest form of olive oil. Research conducted by Menendez J et al. (2013) shows that olive oil is rich in polyphenols. The oil is also known to activate the functioning of the skinny gene which helps you lose weight.

Some other foods you can include in your diet are:

- Green tea
- Citrus fruits
- Blueberries
- Apples
- Medjool dates
- Walnuts
- Turmeric
- Buckwheat
- Parsley
- Soy
- Rocket

Chapter 4:
Juice and Smoothies

Green Juice with Lovage

Serves: 2

Ingredients:

- 4 large handfuls kale leaves, torn
- A handful of lovage leaves
- 1 medium green apple, cored, sliced
- A handful of flat-leaf parsley
- 2 large handfuls of rocket
- 1 teaspoon matcha green tea powder
- Juice of a lemon
- 4 – 6 stalks celery with leaves, chopped

Directions:

1. Juice together kale, parsley, lovage, rocket, apple, and celery in a juicer.

2. Add lemon juice and matcha green tea powder into the extracted juice just before serving.

3. Pour into 2 glasses and serve with ice if desired.

Green Juice with Spinach

Serves: 2

Ingredients:

- 2 large handfuls kale leaves, torn
- 2 large handfuls parsley
- 1 green apple, cored, sliced
- Juice of a lemon
- 2 large handfuls of rocket
- 2 large handfuls of baby spinach
- 1 cucumber, chopped
- 3 inches fresh turmeric, peeled, sliced
- 1 teaspoon matcha green tea powder

Directions:

1. Add kale, parsley lettuce, turmeric, cucumber, apple, and rocket into a juicer and extract the juice.

2. Add lemon juice and matcha green tea powder to the extracted juice just before serving.

3. Pour into 2 glasses and serve with ice.

Sirtfood Wonder Smoothie

Serves: 2

Ingredients:

- 2 handfuls of rocket
- 2 handfuls kale leaves
- 6 sprigs parsley
- 1 handful watercress
- Juice of a lime or lemon
- 1 teaspoon matcha powder
- 1 ½ cups water

Directions:

1. Place all the greens and water in a blender. Blend until smooth.

2. Pour into 2 glasses and serve with ice if desired.

Turmeric Lassi Smoothie

Serves: 2

Ingredients:

- 2 cups frozen mango chunks
- 1 cup low-fat plain Greek yogurt
- ½ inch grated fresh ginger
- ½ tablespoon grated fresh turmeric or ½ teaspoon turmeric powder
- 2 cups ice cubes
- 2 cups water
- 1 cup coconut milk, unsweetened

Directions:

1. Place mango, ginger, turmeric, ginger, and ice cubes in a blender.

2. Pour water, coconut milk, and yogurt.

3. Blend until smooth.

4. Pour into 2 glasses and serve.

Green Smoothie

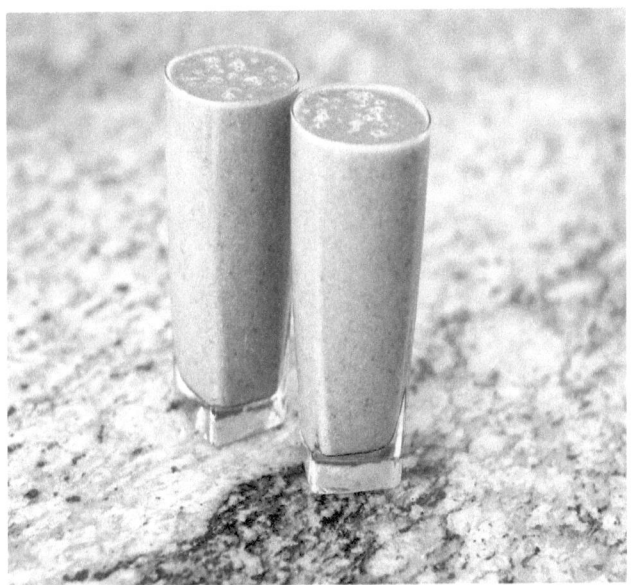

Serves: 2 – 3

Ingredients:

- 1 cup frozen mixed berries
- 1 banana, sliced
- 1 – 2 cups milk of your choice
- 1 cup kale
- 1 cup arugula
- 1 tablespoon ground flaxseeds or chia seeds

Directions:

1. Combine berries, banana, milk, kale, arugula, and flaxseeds in a blender.

2. Blend until you get a nice puree.

3. If you find the smoothie very thick, add some more milk.

4. Pour into glasses and serve.

Chapter 5: Breakfast Recipes

Vegan Buckwheat Banana Bread

Serves: 24

Ingredients:

For Dry Ingredients:

- 3 ½ cups buckwheat flour

- 4 ½ teaspoons baking powder

- 2/3 cup coconut sugar or brown sugar

- ½ teaspoon fine sea salt

- 4 teaspoons ground cinnamon

For wet ingredients:

- 2 teaspoons vanilla extract

- 2/3 cup vegetable oil

- 3 ½ cups very ripe mashed bananas

Directions:

1. Grease 2 loaf pans (9 x 5 inches) with olive oil cooking spray. Place a sheet of parchment paper in each pan. This is optional but helps easy removal of the baked loaves. Also, prepare the oven by preheating it to 350° F.

2. Combine all the dry ingredients in a bowl, i.e., buckwheat flour, baking powder, salt, coconut sugar, and salt.

3. Combine vegetable oil, bananas, and vanilla in another bowl. Whisk until smooth.

4. Pour into the bowl of dry ingredients and stir until just incorporated, making sure not to over mix.

5. Divide the batter among the loaf pans. Place the loaf pans in the oven and bake for about 50 – 55 minutes. To check if the bread is ready, insert a toothpick in the center of the bread. Remove the toothpick. If you see some particles stuck on it, bake for a few more minutes.

Layered Fruit Salad

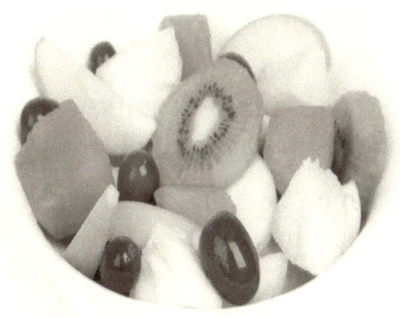

Serves: 3

Ingredients:

- 3 ounces plain nonfat Greek yogurt
- 4 ounces light cream cheese
- ½ teaspoon finely shredded orange zest
- ½ teaspoon finely shredded lemon zest
- 1 ½ kiwifruits, peeled, sliced
- ½ medium orange, peeled, separated into segments, chopped
- ½ cup blueberries
- ½ medium mango, peeled, pitted, cut into cubes
- ½ tablespoon honey

Directions:

1. Place cream cheese in a bowl. Beat with an electric hand mixer set on medium speed until creamy.

2. Add yogurt and beat until well combined. Add honey and beat until smooth.

3. Add lemon zest and orange zest and beat until well combined.

4. Take 3 glasses. Divide equally the fruits among the glasses and place them in layers. Top with cream cheese mixture.

5. Chill until use.

Scrambled Eggs with Mixed Herbs

Serves: 2

Ingredients:

- 4 large eggs
- 1 red onion, chopped
- 2 tablespoons butter
- Flaky sea salt to sprinkle
- ¼ teaspoon coarse salt
- ½ cup chopped flat-leaf parsley
- ½ teaspoon turmeric powder
- Pepper to taste
- Chopped chives to garnish

Directions:

1. Melt butter in a nonstick pan over medium flame. Add onion and sauté until translucent.

2. Add turmeric powder and stir for a few seconds. Crack the eggs in the pan and stir. Sprinkle parsley and stir often until the eggs are soft-cooked.

3. Add salt and pepper to taste and turn off the heat.

4. Garnish with chives and serve.

Buckwheat Porridge

Serves: 4 – 5

Ingredients:

- 4 cups water
- 2 cups buckwheat groats, rinsed

To Serve:

- Cherries
- Milk of your choice
- Vanilla extract
- Ground cinnamon
- Maple syrup or honey
- Walnuts
- Berries

Directions:

1. Cook buckwheat groats with water in a saucepan over medium-high flame. When the mixture comes to a boil, lower the flame and cook covered for about 12 – 13 minutes and not longer. Remove from heat but do not uncover.

2. Let it rest for 5 – 8 minutes.

3. Using a fork, fluff the buckwheat.

4. Divide into bowls. Serve with any one or more of the suggested serving options.

5. Store leftover buckwheat groats in an airtight container in the refrigerator.

Vanilla Chia Seed Pudding

Serves: 4

Ingredients:

- ½ cup chia seeds
- 2 teaspoons vanilla extract
- 4 dates, chopped
- 2 cups almond milk
- 4 walnut halves, chopped
- 4 tablespoons maple syrup

Directions:

1. Combine chia seeds, vanilla, dates, almond milk, walnuts, and maple syrup in a glass bowl.

2. Cover with cling wrap and chill for 3 hours, making sure to stir every hour.

3. Serve.

Chapter 6:
Snack Recipes

Salt and Pepper Roasted Walnuts

Serves: 8 – 10

Ingredients:

- 2 cups walnuts
- Salt to taste
- 2 tablespoons olive oil
- Freshly ground pepper to taste

Directions:

1. Spread the walnuts on a lined baking sheet in a single layer.

2. Roast the walnuts in a preheated oven at 350° F for 8 – 10 minutes or until light brown.

3. Transfer the walnuts to a kitchen towel. Bring the edges of the towel together and rub the walnuts so that the skin comes off.

4. Toss the walnuts with oil, salt, and pepper and spread it back on the baking sheet.

5. Bake for another 2 to 3 minutes.

6. Cool completely and store in an airtight container until use.

Smoked Trout, Arugula, and Granny Smith Stacks

Serves: 8 (2 stacks each)

Ingredients:

- 2 Granny apples, cored, cut each into 8 thin, round slices

- ¾ cup baby arugula leaves

- ½ tablespoon extra-virgin olive oil

- 6 ounces packaged lemon-pepper smoked trout fillets

- 2 tablespoons lemon juice

Directions:

1. Place the apple slices on a serving platter.

2. Flake the fish into smaller pieces after discarding the skin.

3. Place arugula in a bowl. Drizzle oil and lemon juice over it and toss well.

4. Divide the arugula equally and spread it over the apple slices.

5. Divide the fish and place it over the arugula.

6. Serve.

Cinnamon Bun Balls

Serves: 20

Ingredients:

- 10 dates
- 1 cup walnuts
- 6 tablespoons ground cinnamon
- 2 tablespoons finely chopped walnuts
- 2 teaspoons ground cardamom

Directions:

1. Pit the dates and add them into the food processor bowl. Also add walnuts, cardamom, and cinnamon and blend until smooth or the texture you desire is achieved.

2. Transfer the mixture into a bowl. Place chopped walnuts on a plate.

3. Divide the mixture into 20 equal portions and shape it into balls. Moisten your hands with water while making balls. Dredge the balls in chopped walnuts.

4. Transfer the balls into an airtight container. Refrigerate until use. It can last for 7 – 8 days. You can also place it in the freezer. It can last for 3 months in the freezer.

Cranberry Pecan Goat Cheese Balls

Serves: 12 – 15

Ingredients:

For Goat Cheese Balls:

- 3 ounces cream cheese
- 4 ounces goat cheese
- 1 tablespoon honey
- 1 teaspoon ground cinnamon
- ¼ cup finely chopped pecans

For Outer Covering:

- ½ cup finely chopped pecans
- ½ cup diced dried cranberries
- ¼ cup minced fresh parsley

Directions:

1. To make balls: Mix together cream cheese, goat cheese, honey, cinnamon, and pecans in a bowl.

2. Make 12 – 15 small balls of the mixture.

3. To make outer covering: Place cranberries, parsley, and pecans in a bowl and toss well.

4. Dredge the balls in this mixture. Press lightly to adhere. Place the balls on a plate.

5. Dredge the balls once again in the mixture. Press lightly to adhere. Place the balls on a plate.

6. Chill until use. Store leftovers in an airtight container in the refrigerator.

7. Serve as it is or with apple slices or crackers.

Mushroom, Kale, and Buckwheat Muffins

Serves: 20

Ingredients:

- 4 cups sliced mushrooms

- 2 cloves garlic, peeled, minced

- 4 flax eggs (4 tablespoons ground flaxseeds mixed with 12 tablespoons water)

- 1 cup oats

- 2 teaspoons baking soda

- 2 teaspoons dried oregano

- 1 cup almond milk

- Pumpkin seeds, to top

- 4 cups tightly packed kale

- 2 tablespoons fresh thyme

- 2 cups buckwheat flour

- 2 teaspoons baking powder

- 2 teaspoons sea salt

- 2/3 cup olive oil

- 2 tablespoons apple cider vinegar

Directions:

1. Take 2 muffin pans of 12 counts each and line 20 of the muffin molds with disposable liners. Also, prepare the oven by preheating it to 400° F.

2. Place a pan over medium flame. Add oil and let it heat. When the oil is hot, add mushrooms, thyme, and garlic and cook until dry. It should take about 5 minutes.

3. Add kale and stir. Cook until kale wilts. Turn off the heat and let it cool.

4. When you mix together water and ground flaxseed meal, let it rest for 15 minutes. It will be gel-like in 15 minutes.

5. Combine all the dry ingredients in a bowl, i.e., buckwheat flour, baking soda, baking powder, oregano, and salt.

6. Combine almond milk, olive oil, and apple cider vinegar in a bowl. Pour this mixture into the bowl of dry ingredients. Add the flax eggs as well and mix using a wooden spoon until just incorporated, making sure not to over-mix.

7. Add the mushroom mixture and fold gently.

8. Divide the batter into the lined muffin molds. Scatter some pumpkin seeds on top.

9. Place the muffin pans in the oven and bake for about 30 – 35 minutes. To check if the muffins are ready, insert a toothpick in the center of a muffin. Remove the toothpick. If you see some particles stuck on it, bake for a few more minutes.

10. Cool the baked muffins for 10 minutes in the pan itself. Remove muffins from the pan and place on a wire rack to cool completely.

11. Store in an airtight container until use. It can last for 2 – 3 days on your countertop or for 5 – 6 days in the refrigerator.

Chapter 7:
Soup Recipes

Miso Mushroom & Tofu Noodle Soup

Serves: 2

Ingredients:

- 2 tablespoons olive oil
- 3.5 ounces smoked tofu, cut into small pieces
- 3.5 ounces buckwheat noodles
- 2 cups sliced mushrooms
- 1 tablespoon miso paste
- 4 spring onions, thinly sliced
- 3 cups boiling water

Directions:

1. Follow the directions on the package and cook the noodles.

2. Place a pan with 1-tablespoon oil over medium flame. When the oil is heated, add mushrooms and cook until brown.

3. Remove the mushrooms from the pan and place them in a bowl.

4. Pour 1-tablespoon oil into the pan. When the oil is heated, add tofu and cook until brown all over. Turn off the heat.

5. Combine miso paste and boiling water in a bowl.

6. Divide noodles into soup bowls. Scatter mushrooms and tofu over the noodles.

7. Pour miso broth into the bowls. Garnish with spring onions and serve.

Fresh Pea & Lovage Soup

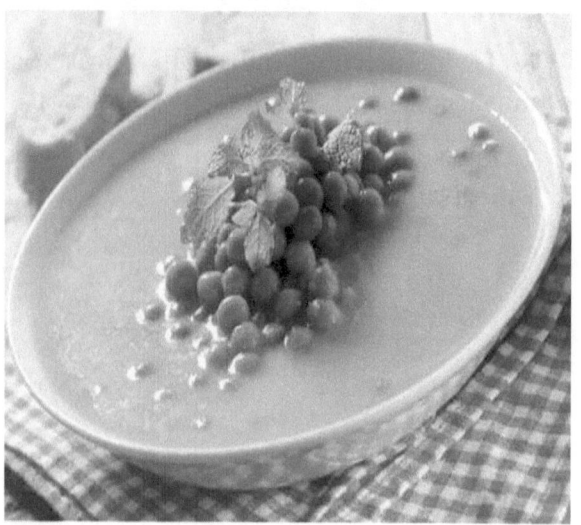

Serves: 4

Ingredients:

- 1 pound frozen peas
- 4 whole pea pods, to garnish
- 2 – 3 spring onions, thinly sliced
- 3 cups vegetable stock
- 5 sprigs lovage, use only the leaves
- 3 tablespoons butter
- Pepper to taste
- 2 small cloves garlic, peeled, finely chopped
- ¼ cup crème fraiche
- Salt to taste

Directions:

1. Place a soup pot over a medium flame. Add butter and let it melt.

2. Add garlic and spring onions and sauté for 3 – 4 minutes.

3. Stir in the broth. When it begins to boil, add peas and whole pods. Cook until peas are soft.

4. Pull out the whole pea pods and rinse under cold water.

5. Add crème fraiche and lovage into the soup and blend with an immersion blender until creamy.

6. Add salt and pepper to taste.

7. You can serve this soup hot or chilled.

8. To serve: Ladle the soup into bowls. Place one whole pod in each bowl.

9. Serve.

German Seven Herb Soup

Serves: 8

Ingredients:

- 2 tablespoons butter
- 2 medium leeks, chopped
- 4 cups chopped spinach
- 2 cups chopped chives
- 2 cups chopped parsley
- 1 cup arugula
- 1 cup chopped fresh dill
- 1 cup chopped celery leaves
- 4 russet potatoes, peeled, cut into cubes
- Freshly ground pepper to taste
- 1 cup milk
- Salt to taste

To Serve: Optional

- Croutons
- Sour cream
- Extra herbs

Directions:

1. Place a soup pot with butter over medium flame. When butter melts, add shallots and leek and sauté until onions are translucent.

2. Stir in potatoes and water and cook until potatoes are soft.

3. Add all the 7 greens and cook for a few minutes until the greens wilt.

4. Turn off the heat. Blend with an immersion blender until creamy.

5. Add salt and pepper to taste. Pour milk and stir.

6. Serve as it is or with suggested serving options.

Turkey Sausage, Butternut Squash & Kale Soup

Serves: 5

Ingredients:

- ½ package (from a 19.5 ounces package) Italian turkey sausage links, discard casings

- 4 cups chicken broth

- ¼ cup shaved parmesan cheese

- 1 ½ pounds butternut squash, peeled, cut into cubes

- Salt to taste

- Pepper to taste

Directions:

1. Place a soup pot over a medium flame. Add sausage and cook until it is not pink anymore. As it cooks, break the sausage into smaller pieces.

2. Add the squash next and mix well. Pour broth and stir. When it comes to a boil, lower the heat and cook until squash is slightly tender.

3. Add kale and cook until it wilts.

4. Ladle into soup bowls. Garnish with parmesan cheese and serve.

Vegetarian Kale Soup

Serves: 4

Ingredients:

- 1 tablespoon olive oil

- 1 tablespoon chopped garlic

- 4 cups water

- ½ can (from a 15 ounces can) diced tomatoes

- 1 can (15 ounces can) cannellini beans, drained

- 1 tablespoon dried parsley

- Salt to taste

- 1 small red onion, chopped

- ½ bunch kale, discard hard stems, chopped

- 3 vegetable bouillon cubes

- 3 white potatoes, peeled, cubed

- ½ tablespoon Italian seasoning

- Pepper to taste

Directions:

1. Place a soup pot over a medium flame. When the oil is hot, add onion and garlic and cook until onion turns translucent.

2. Add kale and stir. Cook for a couple of minutes.

3. Pour water and stir. Crumble bouillon cubes into the pot. Add potatoes, tomatoes, cannellini beans, parsley, and Italian seasoning and stir.

4. When the soup starts boiling, lower the heat and cook covered until potatoes are soft.

5. Add salt and pepper to taste.

Chapter 8: Salad Recipes

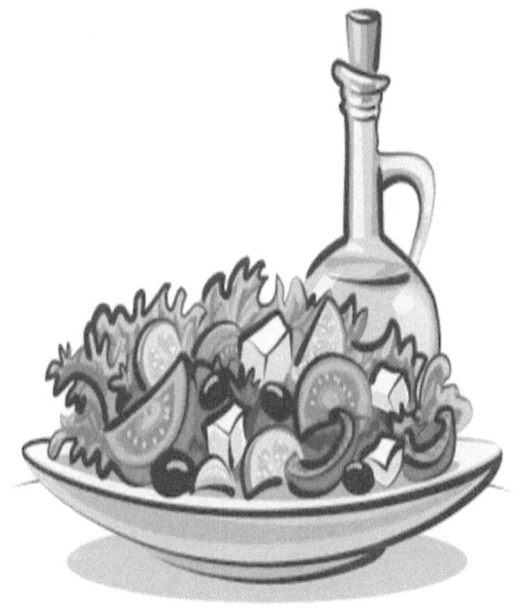

Sirt Super Salad

Serves: 2

Ingredients:

- 3.5 ounces arugula
- 7 ounces smoked salmon slices
- 1 cup chopped celery leaves and stalk
- ½ cup chopped walnuts
- 2 tablespoons extra-virgin olive oil
- 3.5 ounces endive leaves

- 1 cup cubed avocado
- 1 medium red onion, chopped
- 2 tablespoons capers
- ½ cup chopped fresh parsley
- 2 large medjool dates, pitted, chopped
- Juice of ½ lemon

Directions:

1. Add all the greens into a large bowl and toss well.

2. Combine salmon, avocado, capers, walnuts, dates, and red onions in another bowl and toss well.

3. Add lemon juice and oil and toss well.

4. Spread salmon mixture over the greens and serve.

Shredded Brussels Sprouts & Kale Salad

Serves: 3

Ingredients:

For Dressing:

- 2 tablespoons olive oil
- 2 small cloves garlic, minced
- ¼ teaspoon salt
- 3 tablespoons fresh lemon juice
- ½ teaspoon sugar
- Freshly ground pepper to taste

For Salad:

- ½ pound Brussels sprouts, trimmed, discard outer leaves, thinly sliced
- 1 apple, cored, thinly sliced
- 3 tablespoons candied pecans, chopped
- 2 slices cooked turkey bacon, chopped (optional)
- ½ bunch, Tuscan kale, discard stems, thinly slice the leaves
- ¼ cup dried cranberries
- 2 tablespoons crumbled gorgonzola cheese
- Freshly ground pepper to taste

Directions:

1. To make the dressing: Whisk together olive oil, garlic, salt, lemon juice, sugar, and pepper in a small bowl.

2. Combine Brussels sprouts and kale in a bowl. Drizzle dressing over it and toss well. Massage the mixture for a few minutes with your hands until slightly soft.

3. Chill for at least a couple of hours, making sure to cover the bowl while chilling.

4. Add apple slices, turkey bacon, pecans, and cranberries just before serving. Toss well. Sprinkle pepper and Gorgonzola on top and serve.

Apple Pecan Arugula Salad

Serves: 2

Ingredients:

For Salad:

- ¼ cup pecans, toasted

- 1 small apple, cored, peel if desired, cut into thin slices

- 1 tablespoon dried cranberries

- 3.5 ounces arugula

- 1 small red onion, thinly sliced

For Dressing:

- Juice of ½ lemon

- Salt to taste

- Pepper to taste

- ½ tablespoon maple syrup

- 1 ½ tablespoons olive oil

Directions:

1. To make the dressing: Combine lemon juice, salt, pepper, maple syrup, and olive oil in a bowl. Whisk well.

2. To make the salad: Combine apple, cranberries, arugula, and onion in a bowl.

3. Pour dressing over the salad. Toss well.

4. Divide into 2 plates. Garnish with pecans and serve.

Berry and Walnut Salad

Serves: 2

Ingredients:

- 1 ½ tablespoons whole buttermilk
- ½ teaspoon honey
- A pinch pepper
- ½ cup quartered strawberries
- 1 tablespoon chopped, toasted walnuts
- ½ ounce goat cheese softened
- 1/8 teaspoon salt
- 2 cups spring mix
- ¼ cup fresh blueberries

Directions:

1. To make the dressing: Whisk together goat cheese, buttermilk, pepper, salt, and honey in a bowl.

2. Combine strawberries, walnuts, blueberries, and spring mix in another bowl.

3. Pour dressing over the salad. Toss well and serve.

Warm Chicken & Chicory Salad

Serves: 2 – 3

Ingredients:

- 1.8 pounds chicken
- 3. 4 ounces sherry vinegar + ½ tablespoon
- 1 ½ tablespoons olive oil
- A fistful of raisins
- 1 ½ heads chicory
- A fistful pine nuts, toasted
- 2 tablespoons butter, room temperature
- 3.5 ounces frozen peas
- ¼ teaspoon caster sugar
- 1 tablespoon chopped dill
- 1 cup mixed salad leaves
- Salt to taste
- Pepper to taste

Directions:

1. Brush butter all over the chicken. Sprinkle salt and pepper over the chicken and place in a baking pan.

2. Drizzle vinegar all around the chicken. Keep the pan covered with aluminum foil.

3. Bake chicken in a preheated oven at 320° F for about an hour or until cooked through inside.

4. Pour the cooked chicken juices in a bowl and raise the temperature of the oven to 450° F. Do not cover the pan and continue roasting until golden brown on top.

5. Remove the chicken from the oven and let it cool for a few minutes. Shred the chicken with a pair of forks.

6. While the chicken is roasting, pour some water into a saucepan and bring to a boil. Add peas and cook for a minute. Drain off the water and immerse the peas in a bowl of cold water for 10 minutes. Drain once again.

7. In a while, the fat would be floating on top of the cooked juices. Spoon off the fat. Add extra vinegar, caster sugar, and olive oil into the bowl of cooked juices and whisk until sugar dissolves completely.

8. Place roasted chicken, raisins, chicory leaves, salad leaves, pea, and pine nuts in a bowl. Toss well.

9. Pour the cooked liquid over it and toss well.

10. Serve as it is or with some bread of your choice.

Chapter 9:
Side Dish Recipes

Quinoa Kale Stuffing With Squash Rings

Serves: 5

Ingredients:

- 1 small acorn squash (about 1 pound), cut horizontally into 1/8 inch thick slices, deseeded – 5 slices

- Pepper to taste

- Salt to taste

- ½ tablespoon olive oil

For Quinoa Stuffing:

- ½ teaspoon olive oil

- 3 tablespoons diced red or yellow bell pepper

- 10 tablespoons cooked quinoa

- 1/3 cup cooked or canned chickpeas, drained

- 1 small sweet potato, peeled, cut into ½ inch cubes

- ½ cup chopped kale

- Pepper to taste

- 2 tablespoons grated parmesan cheese (optional)

- 1 small shallot, thinly sliced

• Salt to taste

• ½ tablespoon minced fresh oregano or ½ teaspoon dried oregano

Directions:

1. To make stuffing: Pour oil into a skillet and heat over medium flame. Once the oil is hot, add shallot and bell pepper and cook until slightly tender.

2. Stir in sweet potatoes and ¼ cup water and cook until sweet potatoes are fork-tender.

3. Add quinoa and mix well. Heat thoroughly.

4. Stir in the kale, chickpeas, parmesan if using, salt and pepper, and mix well. Heat thoroughly. Once kale wilts, turn off the heat.

5. Line a baking sheet with parchment paper. Place the squash rings on the baking sheet without overlapping. Place about ½ cup of quinoa on each slice of squash.

6. Bake squash with stuffing in an oven that has been preheated 425° F for about 15 minutes or until squash is slightly tender or not mushy.

Veggie Stir Fry

Serves: 4

Ingredients:

- 4 teaspoons olive oil
- 2 2/3 cups cauliflower florets
- 2 2/3 cups broccoli florets
- 2 2/3 cups carrot slices, cut at a slight angle
- ½ teaspoon minced ginger
- ½ teaspoon minced garlic
- 4 teaspoons soy sauce
- 2/3 cup chicken broth
- 2 teaspoons cornstarch mixed with 2 tablespoons water

Directions:

1. Place a nonstick pan over a medium-high flame. Add oil and let it heat. When the oil is heated, add ginger, garlic, and vegetables and stir-fry for a couple of minutes.

2. Stir in broth and simmer for a few minutes until vegetables are crisp as well as tender.

3. Add soy sauce and cornstarch and constantly stir until thick. Turn off the heat and serve.

Crispy Turmeric Roasted Potatoes

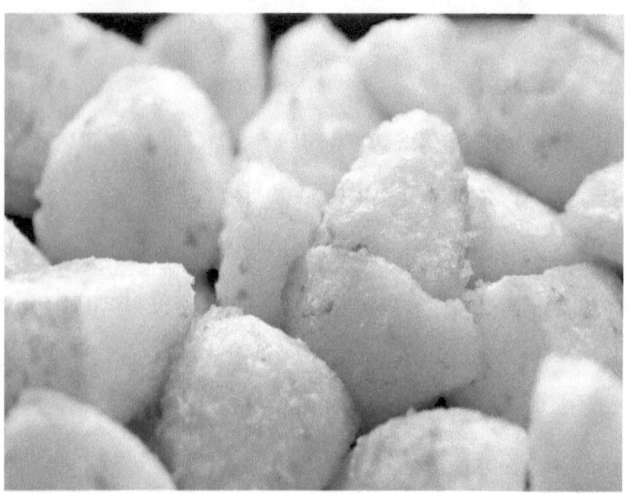

Serves: 3

Ingredients:

- 1 small red onion, chopped
- 2 ½ cups cubed potatoes
- ½ teaspoon salt
- 1 teaspoon curry powder (optional)
- 2 cloves garlic, minced
- 1 teaspoon turmeric powder
- Pepper to taste
- 2 tablespoons olive oil

Directions:

1. Place garlic, onion, and potatoes in a bowl and toss well. Sprinkle salt, turmeric, curry powder, pepper, and olive oil and toss well. Drizzle oil and stir until well combined.

2. Line a baking sheet with parchment paper.

3. Spread the potatoes on the baking sheet.

4. Bake potatoes in an oven that has been preheated 375° F for about 35 minutes or until potatoes are fork-tender. Stir the potatoes every 10 – 12 minutes.

Sunshine Salad

Serves: 4

Ingredients:

- 8 cups thinly sliced spinach

- 2 cups sliced strawberries

- 4 tablespoons roasted sunflower seeds

- 2 oranges, peeled, separated into segments, deseeded, chopped

- ½ cup light or low-calorie Italian dressing or raspberry vinaigrette

Directions:

1. Place spinach, strawberries, and oranges in a bowl and toss well.

2. Add dressing and stir until well combined.

3. Garnish with sunflower seeds and serve.

Parsley & Caper Salad

Serves: 4

Ingredients:

- 2 cups chopped flat-leaf parsley leaves

- ½ cup finely chopped flat-leaf parsley stems

- 2 tablespoons capers, drained, finely chopped

- 3 tablespoons olive oil

- 2 Little Gem lettuces, separate the leaves

- Juice of ½ lemon

- ¼ shallot, finely chopped

- Salt to taste

- 1 cup halved cherry tomatoes

Directions:

1. To make the dressing: Combine olive oil, parsley stalks, capers, lemon juice, and shallot in a bowl.

2. Add parsley leaves, tomatoes, and lettuce and toss well.

3. Serve right away.

Chapter 10:
Lunch / Dinner Recipes

Raw Rainbow Collard Greens Wrap

Serves: 8

Ingredients:

- 8 large collard leaves, rinsed

- 2 tomatoes, cut into thin wedges

- 2 yellow bell peppers, cut into thin strips

- 1 cup pea sprouts

- ¼ head red cabbage, shredded

- 2 medium carrots, cut into matchsticks

- 1 Persian cucumbers, cut into matchsticks

- ½ red onion, cut into thin strips

- 1 ½ cups hummus

- 1 teaspoon grated horseradish in beet juice

Directions:

1. Place the collard green leaves on your cutting board, with the rib side up. Carefully cut thin slices the ribs off the leaves so that they are flat. Do this with all the leaves.

2. Spread hummus on the leaves. Divide all the vegetables among the leaves and keep the leaves parallel to the spine, leaving the borders.

3. Spoon some horseradish over the vegetables.

4. Fold like burritos and place on a serving platter, with the seam side down.

Avocado Chickpea Lettuce Wraps

Serves: 2

Ingredients:

- ½ can (from a 15 ounces can) chickpeas, drained
- 1 stalk celery, finely chopped
- ½ tablespoon lemon juice
- 2 Boston lettuce leaves
- ½ ripe avocado, peeled, pitted, chopped
- 1 green onion, finely chopped
- Salt to taste
- Pepper to taste

For Toppings:

- Alfalfa sprouts
- Chopped tomatoes
- Cucumber, cut into matchsticks
- Bell pepper strips
- Chopped parsley

Directions:

1. Place chickpeas and mash them until you are left with a few chunks.

2. Add avocado and mash to the desired texture.

3. Stir in salt, pepper, onion, celery, and lemon juice.

4. Spread the lettuce leaves on a plate. Divide the filling among the leaves. Place suggested toppings. Roll and serve.

Cauliflower Kale Frittata

Serves: 4

Ingredients:

- 2 cups grated or finely chopped cauliflower
- 4 large eggs
- 12 large egg whites
- 2 tablespoons milk
- 2 cups shredded kale leaves, discard hard ribs and stems
- ½ teaspoon garlic powder
- 3 teaspoons grated parmesan cheese
- ½ cup water
- Pepper to taste
- 1 teaspoon dried thyme
- Salt to taste
- Olive oil cooking spray

Directions:

1. Place a cast-iron skillet over a medium-high flame.

2. When the skillet is well heated, add cauliflower to the pan. Pour water and cook until tender.

3. Meanwhile, whisk together eggs, whites, salt, pepper, and milk in a bowl with an

electric hand mixer until frothy, at least 2 – 3 minutes.

4. Add garlic powder, kale, and thyme into the skillet and stir. Once the kale wilts, turn off the heat.

5. Remove the vegetables from the pan and place them in the bowl of the egg mixture. Stir well.

6. Place the skillet back over medium flame. Spray the skillet with cooking spray. Let the pan heat.

7. Pour the egg mixture into the skillet. Do not stir now.

8. Scatter parmesan cheese on top. Cover the skillet with a lid. Cook for a few minutes. When the edges look set, turn off the heat.

9. Set up your oven to broil mode. Place the rack 6 inches below the heating element and preheat the oven to high heat.

10. Transfer the skillet into the oven and broil without covering until it sets in the middle. It should take 7 – 10 minutes.

11. Remove the skillet from the oven and let it cool for 5 minutes. Cut into 4 equal wedges.

12. Serve hot or warm.

Coffee Rubbed Burgers

Serves: 8

Ingredients:

- 2 pounds lean ground turkey
- 4 teaspoons brown sugar
- 2 teaspoons red pepper flakes, finely ground
- 1 teaspoon garlic salt
- 1 teaspoon onion powder
- 2 tablespoons ground coffee beans
- 4 teaspoons freshly ground pepper
- 1 teaspoon dry mustard powder
- ½ teaspoon ground cloves
- 1 teaspoon unsweetened cocoa powder

Directions:

1. Divide ground turkey into 8 equal portions and shape into patties.

2. Place onion powder, ground coffee beans, pepper, mustard powder, cloves, and cocoa in a Ziploc plastic bag. Seal the bag and shake the bag until well combined.

3. Sprinkle a generous amount of the mixture all over the burgers. Rub it into it.

4. Cook the burgers either in a pan or in an oven or grill and serve with toppings of your choice.

Roasted Chicken Breast with Walnuts, Dates, and Olives

Serves: 3

Ingredients:

- 3 boneless chicken breast halves
- 1/3 cup red wine vinegar
- 6 tablespoons toasted, chopped walnuts
- 6 – 7 tablespoons chicken stock
- A handful Italian parsley, chopped
- 3 – 4 Medjool dates, pitted, chopped
- 1 tablespoon olive oil
- Salt to taste
- 3 tablespoons pitted, sliced olives
- 2 teaspoons butter
- Pepper to taste

Directions:

1. Soak dates in vinegar for a couple of hours.

2. Place an ovenproof skillet over a medium-high flame. Add oil and let it heat. Add chicken cook until brown all over. Turn off the heat and shift the skillet into an oven that has been preheated to 325° F. Cook for about 12 – 15 minutes or until chicken is cooked through.

3. Place a skillet over a high flame. Pour the stock into the skillet. Add walnuts, dates along

with vinegar and olives and let it come to a boil.

4. Stir in parsley and butter. Add salt and pepper to taste. Pour this sauce over the chicken and serve.

Beef and Red Wine Stew

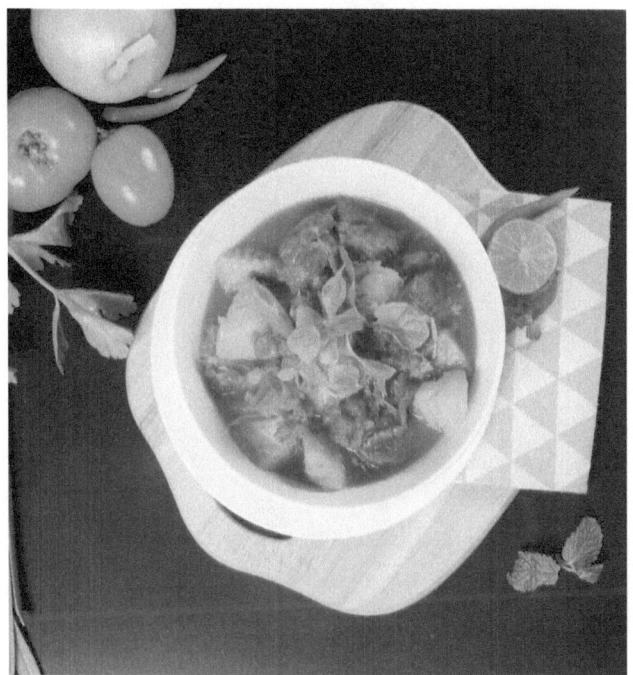

Serves: 3

Ingredients:

- 1 tablespoon butter
- 3 cloves garlic, peeled, halved
- 1.1 pounds beef skirt or shin, chopped into large pieces
- 1 tablespoon olive oil
- 2 small cloves garlic, crushed
- A handful chopped fresh flat-leaf parsley

- 2 sprigs thyme + extra to serve, finely chopped

- 2 sprigs rosemary + extra to serve, finely chopped

- 2 tablespoons seasoned flour

- 6 ounces beef stock

- 2 tablespoons tomato puree

- 1 large onion, diced

- 6.3 ounces red wine

- Salt to taste

- Pepper to taste

- Mashed potatoes to serve (optional)

Directions:

1. Place a heatproof casserole dish over a medium flame. Pour ½ tablespoon olive oil and let it heat.

2. Place flour in a plastic bag. Place beef in the bag and shake the bag until beef pieces are well coated with the flour.

3. When the oil is heated, add beef and cook until beef is brown on all the sides. Remove beef with a slotted spoon and place on a plate.

4. Add ½ tablespoon olive oil and let it heat. Add onion and garlic and sauté until soft. Add stock and tomato puree and stir.

5. Add red wine and scrape the bottom of the dish to remove any browned bits.

6. When it begins to boil, turn off the heat. Close the casserole dish with its lid. Shift the casserole dish into an oven that has been preheated to 300° F. Cook for about 45 – 50 minutes.

7. Stir in mushrooms and cover the dish. Continue baking until meat is tender. Garnish with parsley and serve.

Miso Marinated Cod with Stir-Fried Greens & Sesame

Serves: 2

Ingredients:

- 2 ½ tablespoons miso or more to taste
- 2 tablespoons extra-virgin olive oil
- 1 medium red onion, sliced
- 2 cloves garlic, peeled, finely chopped
- 2 teaspoons minced ginger
- 3.5 ounces kale, chopped
- A handful parsley, chopped
- 2.1-ounce buckwheat
- 2 tablespoons mirin
- 14.1 ounces skinless cod fillets
- 2 stalks celery, sliced
- 2 bird's eye chilies, finely chopped
- 4 ounces green beans, trimmed, cut into 2-inch pieces
- 2 teaspoons sesame seeds
- 2 tablespoons tamari
- 2 teaspoons ground turmeric

Directions:

1. Combine mirin, miso, and 2 teaspoons olive oil in a bowl. Rub this mixture over the cods. Place the cod in a baking pan. Let it rest for 30 minutes.

2. Follow the directions on the package and cook the buckwheat. Add turmeric while cooking the buckwheat.

3. Bake the cos in a preheated oven at 450° F for 10 minutes.

4. Place a large pan over medium flame. Add remaining oil and let it heat. Add onion once the oil is hot and cook for a couple of minutes.

5. Stir in celery, bird's eye chilies, green beans, ginger, garlic, and kale, and cook until veggies are tender. Sprinkle some water if required.

6. Stir in sesame seeds, tamari, and parsley.

7. Divide the stir-fry into 2 plates. Divide the cod among the plates and serve.

Bean and Buckwheat Stew

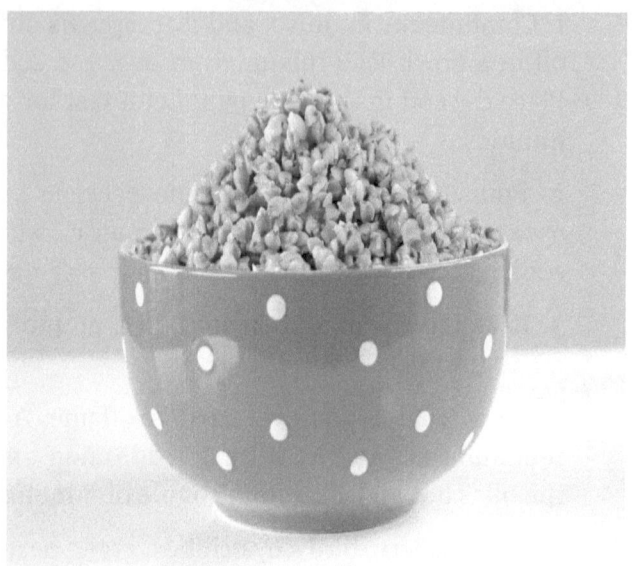

Serves: 8

Ingredients:

- 4 tablespoons olive oil
- 4 carrots, cut into small cubes
- 2 large leeks, chopped
- 2 tablespoons tomato puree
- 2 cans (15 ounces each) cannellini beans or any other beans of your choice
- 2 cloves garlic, crushed
- 4 sticks celery, chopped
- 7 – 8 cups vegetable stock

• 6 tablespoons buckwheat

• 1 bird's eye chili, sliced

• 2 cups chopped kale or any other greens of your choice

• Chopped parsley to garnish

Directions:

1. Place a soup pot over a medium flame. Pour oil and let it heat. Once the oil is hot, add garlic and stir for 5 – 6 seconds. Stir in celery, carrots, and leeks and cook until slightly tender.

2. Mix in tomato puree, stock, and buckwheat. When it comes to a boil, lower the heat and cook until buckwheat is tender.

3. Stir in beans and greens and simmer for a few more minutes, until the greens wilt.

4. Serve.

Chapter 11:
Dessert Recipes

Chocolate Covered Date Nut Bars

Serves: 12

Ingredients:

- ½ cup pitted, packed medjool dates
- 3 ounces dark chocolate chips
- ¾ cup walnuts

Directions:

1. Prepare a small baking sheet or pan by lining it with parchment paper.

2. Soak dates in a bowl of hot water for 5 minutes. Drain and add into the food processor bowl.

3. Add walnuts and process until walnuts are finely chopped, and the mixture should stick together when pressed together.

4. Spread the mixture on the baking sheet. Press it well.

5. Melt chocolate in a microwave or double boiler and drizzle all over the walnut mixture. The whole mixture should be covered with chocolate, so spread it with a spoon if necessary.

6. Freeze for 10 minutes or until chocolate sets.

7. Cut into 12 equal bars and serve.

8. Store leftovers in an airtight container in the refrigerator.

Strawberry-Rhubarb Cobbler with Granola Streusel

Serves: 8

Ingredients:

For Topping:

- 1 cup old-fashioned oats

- 1 cup lightly packed brown sugar

- 8 tablespoons unsalted butter, melted

- 2/3 cup whole-wheat flour or buckwheat flour

- 2 teaspoons ground cinnamon (optional)

For Filling:

- 8 tablespoons pure maple syrup or granulated sugar

- 6 cups sliced rhubarb, fresh or frozen (thaw if frozen)

- 6 cups quartered strawberries

- 2 tablespoons lemon juice

- 2 tablespoons cornstarch

- ½ teaspoon salt

Directions:

1. Grease a baking dish with some olive oil cooking spray. You need to preheat your oven to 350° F for 15 – 20 minutes.

2. Combine strawberries, rhubarb, honey, salt, lemon juice, and cornstarch in a bowl. Toss until well combined. Spoon the mixture into the baking dish.

3. To make topping: Combine oats, cinnamon, brown sugar, and flour in a bowl. Add butter and mix well. Scatter this mixture all over the berry mixture.

4. Pop the baking dish in the oven and bake for about 50 minutes until the top is brown

5. Take out the baking dish from the oven and let it cool on your countertop for 15 minutes before serving.

Stuffed Dates

Serves: 10

Ingredients:

- 10 dates
- 1 tablespoon honey
- 2 – 3 tablespoons goat cheese

Directions:

1. Take out the pit from the dates, carefully; making sure you slit only one side while removing the pit.

2. Combine honey and goat cheese in a bowl. Fill this mixture in the dates and serve.

Frozen Blueberry Coconut Yogurt Pie

Serves: 16

Ingredients:

- 2 cups toasted coconut

- 2 cups fresh blueberries

- 6 cups vanilla Greek yogurt

- 2 prepared graham cracker pie crusts

Directions:

1. Place coconut and yogurt in a bowl and stir. Spread this mixture over the piecrusts. Scatter blueberries on top.

2. Cover and freeze for 6 – 7 hours. Cut each into 8 wedges and serve.

Matcha Ice Cream

Serves: 6

Ingredients:

- 6 bananas, sliced, frozen

- 2 tablespoons matcha powder

- ½ cup coconut cream

- Dark chocolate chips or chopped walnuts, as required

Directions:

1. Combine matcha powder and coconut cream in a bowl and chill for a minimum of 3 hours.

2. Add banana slices and cream cheese mixture into a blender and blend until you get soft-serve consistency.

3. Garnish with chocolate chips and walnuts and serve.

Conclusion

If you are keen to switch to a new lifestyle or eating pattern, the Sirtfood diet is the right one for you. This diet has gained immense popularity in the last few years, and rightfully so. The Sirtfood diet does not focus on excluding any food from the diet because of which you do not feel deprived of the food you enjoy. The diet relies on the ingredients, which improve your health and help you maintain your health. You can also meet your weight loss and fitness goals.

When you begin this diet, your sleep patterns move, lose weight, and regulate and manage your appetite easily. The diet also enhances your immunity and improves your mood. This diet is split into two phases, and you can repeat these steps as often as you want to until you meet your fitness and weight loss goals.

This book has everything you need to learn about the Sirtfood diet. You will learn what the Sirtfood diet is and its benefits. You will also learn more about how the diet works and the foods you should include in your diet if you want to reap its benefits. I am sure you know the diet is easy to follow, and you do not have to compromise on your lifestyle to follow this diet. The book also has numerous Sirtfood diet recipes you can use to start with this diet.

As with every other diet, you should learn to be patient with your body. It is important to understand that your body will take some time to adapt to changes in your diet and lifestyle. If you combine this diet with exercise, you can reap the benefits of this diet. So, what are you waiting for? Take the plunge and change your lifestyle now.